LOVE YOUR LIVER

How to Keep Your Liver Healthy

PENNY LANE

We encourage all readers to see a licensed physician or nutritionist if they have any concerns regarding health issues related to diet. Neither the author nor publisher of this eBook takes responsibility for any possible consequences from following any of these recipes. Always speak with your primary health care provider before engaging in any form of self-treatment.

TABLE OF CONTENTS

GOOD DIET TO AID THE LIVER 27

RECIPES GOOD FOR THE LIVER 30

Salmon with walnut 44

Spinach pie 45

Vegetable curry 47

Savoury Rissoles 49

Chicken risotto 50

Easy Tarragon Chicken 53

DESSERTS 54

Custard with Baked apples 54

Apple crumble 56

RECAP; 58

THE LIVER

The health of the liver cannot be under estimated. It is the largest organ in the body, weighing about 1.5kg in an adult and performs some 500 jobs which includes at the minimum 22 vital functions. Some function or malfunction of this organ can be traced in almost every disease. The liver is the chemical factory of the body. When liver damage occurs it results in toxins escaping into the body, which is often the forerunner of many diseases and especially cancer. A second cause of many diseases is the poor quality of the food we habitually eat in the western world.

Many primitive peoples, living simply on food they have hunted or grown, have been found to be virtually free from cancer, heart disease, high blood pressure and obesity. An alteration takes place when they change to a western diet.

Signs of a liver disorder are a feeling of heaviness or discomfort on the right side, a general sluggishness and tiredness for no obvious reason.

Innumerable toxins are constantly assailing the body. The air breathed in urban industrial areas contains many pollutants, far more than air in rural environments.

The poisons in many beverages may include flavorings, sweeteners, preservatives, coloring, anti oxidants, caffeine and stabilizers in soft drinks, and additives of various kinds in alcoholic drinks. Plain tap water can contain chemicals such as chlorine, fluoride, bleach, detergents and more. Many soft drinks contribute to liver disease, in addition to harming the teeth and contributing nothing to the nutrition of the body.

In commercial foods there are many hazards presented. These are; possible residues of artificial fertilizers and herbicides, antibiotics, and synthetic hormones fed to cattle and poultry, mercury in fish, innumerable chemicals added to prolong the shelf life, flavor, color and texture. Many of the food additives have been found on test animals, to either cause damage to the liver or to be carcinogenic, capable of causing cancer.

Although the liver has an amazing ability to regenerate itself, the effects of persistent and long-term alcohol abuse may cause liver failure.

PROTECT YOUR LIVER

The liver must be protected from these chemicals by avoiding as many as possible. Choose foods as close to their natural state as possible. Have a wide range of fresh fruits, salads and vegetables, whole grains, and adequate protein as possible. Stay away from synthetic beverages, tinned, microwaved and processed foods.

Use methods of preparation which retain most or all of the natural goodness and flavor, avoiding over cooking.

TEN TIPS FOR GOOD LIVER HEALTH

1) Keep your weight healthy

Of people diagnosed as obese, about 30% will have fatty livers. This puts them at a higher risk of scarring of the liver (cirrhosis), liver cancer and liver failure. Exercising regularly and eating food that are high in fiber and low in fats will help the liver. Anti-oxidants, minerals and vitamins rich food will also aid you in maintaining a healthy liver and weight.

2) Fad diets -Avoid

Fad diets can cause your weight to yo-yo and put excessive strain on the liver. Try to drop weight healthily by losing about 1-2lbs a week (½ -1kg.)

3) Lower your fat consumption.

High fat levels of the blood and high of cholesterol levels are common contributors to fat liver disease.

4) Moderate your alcohol intake.

Alcohol is toxic to the liver and moderation of alcohol intake is vital for your health.

5) Have blood tests regularly

Having regular blood tests is the key to keeping a check on the cholesterol, fat, and glucose levels of your blood and the health of your liver.

6) Stop smoking

Smoking cigarettes creates toxins in the body and is linked to liver cancer.

7) Had a jab?

Ask your doctor's advice about having a vaccine against A and B hepatitis. If you decide not to have a hepatitis A vaccine, avoid sushi, oysters, scallops, mussels or partially cooked or raw clams. These seafoods frequently live in seas and rivers contaminated with hepatitis A. If you forgo the hepatitis B vaccines practice safer sex.

8) Check with your doctor

The mixing of medications should never be done without advice from a qualified pharmacist or doctor. This advice is relevant to herbal medicines and supplements and also to those bought in the pharmacy and prescription drugs. Many medications need the liver to work harder to metabolize them, and mixing medications can cause damage to the liver. A few herbal supplements are toxic to the liver, herbal supplements such as comfrey, kava, and kombucha tea.

9) Drug risk awareness

Some illegal drugs are cut with chemicals that can be extremely toxic for the liver. Drug use intravenously is known to sometimes spread hepatitis B and C. Don't ever share needles.

10) Exercise Regularly.

FOODS TO AVOID

These foods have been found to contribute to congestion, fatty infiltration, increased cholesterol, and are lacking in essential nutrients.

Animal Fats

Refined Carbohydrates — white flour, white sugar

Processed foods containing additives (preservatives, colorings, flavourings, stabilizers, emulsifiers,)

Vinegar, pickles, highly spiced food

Chocolate

Dairy Products

FOOD TO BE ENJOYED IN ABUNDANCE

All Salads-fresh and organically grown when possible.

All Vegetables-fresh and organically grown when possible. Taken raw when possible in juices.

All Fruits-raw when suitable.

FOODS ESPECIALLY BENEFICIAL TO THE LIVER

Foods good for the liver can be divided into two categories -foods which contains high amount of antioxidants and secondly foods that encourage the detoxification process of the liver.

1. Garlic

Garlic is considered by many to be a miracle herb. It activates liver enzymes that aid the body in flushing out toxins. It also suppresses cholesterol production in the liver. Garlic contains high amounts of selenium, and allicin a natural ingredient that fights infection. Both natural substances that help in liver cleansing.

2. Grapefruit

Grapefruits are high in antioxidants and vitamin C, grapefruit aids the natural cleaning process of the liver. A glass of fresh grapefruit juice helps increase liver detoxifying enzymes that aid in flushing out carcinogens and various other toxins.

3. Carrots

It contains Beta-carotene which is a potent antioxidant. They also contain the vitamins B, C, D, E and K, as well as potassium, sodium, calcium and zinc

4. Beetroot

Good source of potassium contains vitamins C, B and trace minerals. Eating both carrots and beets helps stimulate and improve general liver functions. The combination makes a very good juice.

5. Green Tea

Green tea is full of healthy plant antioxidants and aids the general functions of the liver.

6. Green Leafy Vegetables

Green leafy vegetables may be eaten cooked, raw or juiced. They help eliminate from the blood stream environmental toxins.

7. Avocados

Avocadoes are full of nutrients that aid the body in producing glutathione, this is a substance that is necessary in the livers work of fighting harmful toxins.

8. Apples

A fresh apple is an excellent healthy snack. They contain vitamins A,B and C along with pectin and other elements required by the body to clean and eliminate toxins from the body. They may also help in the treatment of diarrhea and constipation.

9. Olive Oil

Organic oils that are cold-pressed like flax-seed olive, and hemp are good for the liver, provided you use them in moderation. They aid the body by sucking up harmful toxins.

10. Whole Grains

Grains such as brown rice are rich sources of B vitamins. They are known to improve metabolization of fat, liver decongestion and liver function.

11.Cruciferous Vegetables

These vegetables are excellent for the body and increase the production of enzymes in the liver. These aid the liver in flushing out toxins, and carcinogens, which lowers the risk of cancer.

12. Lemons & Limes

Lemons and limes contain large amounts of vitamin C. Lemon juice contains an oil that stimulates the liver to expel toxins from the body.

Drinking a glass of freshly-squeezed lemon or lime juice in the morning is a great way to start the day by stimulating the liver.

14. Turmeric

Is known to be excellent for the liver. It helps relieves digestive problems and calm inflammation. It also helps with circulation and has an anti-bacterial action. It aids enzymes in flushing out carcinogens.

VITAMINS AND MINERALS TO AID THE LIVER

Vitamin C

This vitamin is essential, it protects the liver, is anti-allergic, aids healing and recovery from tiredness.

Vitamin A

Vitamin A builds up protection from toxins and helps with the detoxification of a sluggish liver. It also aids in promoting organ function and healthy skin. Vitamin A is found in foods like beets, carrots, leafy green vegetables, fish and eggs and most fruits.

Vitamin E

Vitamin E protects against environmental poisons and is needed to protect Vitamin A. The two Vitamins combined make a powerful liver tonic. Vitamin E also reduces the need for oxygen in the tissues.

Vitamin E is present in many foods such as avocados, cold-pressed vegetable oils, sunflower seeds, almonds, walnuts, and green vegetables.

B-vitamins

B-vitamins such as B5, B6,B12and

folic acid all aid liver health. These vitamins enable the liver to work more effectively. To make a difference, a person must eat foods that contain B-vitamins. B-vitamins can be found in almonds,bananas, fish, poultry, avocadoes, cheese, pine nuts, sesame seeds, brewer's yeast and brown rice.

<u>Vitamin D</u>

Vitamin D reduces inflammation in the body. Vitamin D is present in eggs, milk, fatty fish such as herring, salmon and tuna and bread.

<u>Vitamin K</u>

Vitamin K is vital for the blood-coagulating factor produced in the liver. It is present in many fresh vegetables, especially curly kale, swiss chard, spinach, broccoli, brussel sprouts and spring onions.

JUICES FOR THE LIVER

Beet & Carrot Juice

5-6 scrapped and cleaned carrots

4-5 small beets

One of the best detoxifying juices especially for the kidneys.

Carrot, celery, cucumber & beet juice

2 carrots

1beet

1 celery stick

1 cucumber

A fantastic breakfast drink that is highly effective in cleansing the liver.

Citrus blend

1 lemon

3 oranges

½ a grapefruit

If too bitter add a teaspoon of honey. Another good breakfast juice.

Cabbage juice

2 pears

1/4 small cabbage

3 celery sticks

Handful of watercress

Raw cabbage juice can taste rather sharp but it helps digestion and also prevents constipation and fluid retention. Cabbages contain compounds that aid the liver to function well and protect against cancer. Watercress, celery and pears are also intestinal cleansers and help to detox the liver.

Wheatgrass juice

Wheatgrass has levels of chlorophyll which work as a natural antiseptic, neutralize toxins and can cleanse the body.

Super Green

4 celery sticks

2 cucumbers

2 handfuls of spinach

1 Handful lettuce leaves

1 Handful of kale

Parsley Sprigs

TIP: It is best to add the cucumbers and celery last, as these will help flush the fibers of the other greens from the juicer.

Fruit liver cleanse

4 apples

1 bunch seedless grapes

2 beets

1/2 grapefruit

1/2 lemon

Carrot & Apple cleanser

6 carrots

3 apples

1/2 lemon

Handful of dandelion leaves

Alkaline liver cleanse

2 grapefruits

4 lemons

2 grated cloves of garlic.

2 inches of ginger-grated.

2 Tbs flax oil

Dash of cayenne

Juice the grapefruit and the lemon before adding the other ingredients.

Contributes to the building of red blood cells, is cleansing and is good in liver and gall bladder conditions.

Grape Juice Liver Cleanse

Ingredients

500 ml Boiled Water – allowed to cool

6 Fresh lemons

Ginger root

3 Grapefruits

3 tbsp Flaxseed oil

6 Garlic cloves

3 to 4 pinches Cumin powder

4 to 6 Fresh Mint leaves

STEPS;

1. Squeeze the grape fruit and lemon and put aside.

2. In the blender, add grated ginger, garlic and some water.

3. Liquidize well.

4. Add the two juices and blend the mixture with the cumin powder and flaxseed oil for 50 seconds.

5. Pour the juice into a glass, garnish

with mint leaves and serve.

The cumin powder and flaxseed oil aid in flushing out harmful toxins out of the liver.

Detox Vegetable Juice

Ingredients

125 g Fresh cabbage

1 Fresh lemon

25g Celery

2 Fresh pears

Ginger root

500 ml Filtered Water

5to 6 Fresh Mint leaves

STEPS;

1. Chop the cabbage, pear, ginger, and celery into small pieces and put in a blender. Add a cup of water.

2. Blend for 11/2 minutes.

3. Add to the blender the fresh lemon juice.

4. Pour the blended juice into a glass

and serve cold with mint leaves.

Annie's Liver Cleanser

Ingredients

300 ml Distilled water

2 grapefruits

2 tbsp cold pressed flax oil

4 Lemons

2 inches Fresh ginger root

4 cloves Fresh garlic

1 tsp Acidophilus (a probiotic)

Cayenne pepper (add to taste)

STEPS;

1. Juice the grape fruit and lemon and put in the blender.

2. Chop the garlic and ginger and add to blender.

3. Add water and acidophilus powder and blend for 50 seconds.

Pour the mixture into a glass and add cayenne pepper to taste.

GOOD DIET TO AID THE LIVER

1st thing in the morning;

Small tumbler of fresh diluted fruit juice ie apple, pineapple, lemon or grapefruit with equal quantity of water.

Breakfast

Fresh Fruit; apple, pear, grapes, grapefruit or other fruit as available.

Muesli with one tablespoon each of wheat germ, raisins, sunflower seeds, and milled nuts, moistened with fruit juice or a little milk.

Or

Porridge with one or two slices of whole wheat toast.

Mid-morning

Diluted vegetable or fruit juice.

Lunch

A small glassful of grapefruit or

apple juice, sipped slowly.

A good mixed salad, chosen from: lettuce, rocket lettuce, watercress, endive, Chinese leaves, shredded raw cabbage, tomato, radish, cucumber, celery, spring onion, Spanish Onion, chopped fennel, grated raw carrot, grated raw beetroot, parsley, chives, sage (or other fresh herbs chopped), cottage cheese, dates, walnut, nuts and raisins.

Whole-wheat crisp bread or baked jacket potato.

Afternoon

Herb tea, fruit juice or vegetable juice

Dinner

Small glassful of vegetable or fruit juice, melon or homemade vegetable soup.

A protein dish: ie Easy Tarragon Chicken

Ingredients;

1 Chicken

2 tbsps unsalted butter

1 tbsp chopped fresh tarragon

1 clove garlic, chopped

Sea salt and black pepper

Olive oil

STEPS;

- Preheat oven to 200°C
- Clean and trim chicken
- Mix together the butter, tarragon, garlic and seasoning
- Place the mixture into the cavity of the chicken secure with a cocktail stick
- Rub the skin of the chicken with olive oil.
- Place the chicken upside down in a roasting tin and toast for 1 ¼-1 ½ hours basting at intervals.
- Serve with a mixed green salad and a vegetable of your choice lightly steamed.

RECIPES GOOD FOR THE LIVER

STARTERS

Borsch (beetroot soup)

Ingredients

2¼lb (1kg) beetroot

1lb (450g) carrots

4 onions

2 roughly chopped garlic cloves,

2 roughly chopped sticks of celery,

1 bay leaf

1 1/2 tbsp caraway seeds

Vegetable Stock

salt and freshly ground black pepper

STEPS;

1.	Peel and roughly slice the vegetables. Put in a large saucepan with the caraway seeds and bay leaf.

2. Cover all with the vegetable stock.

3. Bring to the boil. Cover the saucepan and simmer until the vegetables are tender (about 1 hour.)

3. Remove the bay leaf.

4. Pour the soup into a blender and liquidize the soup until smooth.

5 Adjust the seasoning.

6. Reheat gently, serve with soured cream.

In the summer this soup can be enjoyed cold.

Potato, Carrot and Pumpkin soup

Serves: 6

Ingredients

1 small peeled pumpkin chopped

2 medium carrots, peeled and chopped

2 large potatoes, peeled and chopped

1 onion, chopped

4 sliced garlic cloves,

2 chicken stock cubes dissolved in 1 litre of hot water

1 vegetable stock cube dissolved in 2 tablespoons of boiling water

1 tspoon curry paste

Black pepper

2 tblsps cream

1 tblsps olive oil

STEPS;

1. In a saucepan, put the onion and garlic and cook gently in the olive oil until

soft.

2. Add in the curry paste, stir and continue cooking for 2 minutes.

3. Add the vegetables and chicken stock, and bring to the boil

4. Cover with a lid and gently simmer until the ingredients are tender.

5. Cool

6. Adjust seasoning and liquidize the soup.

7. Add the cream

Vegetable soup

Serves: 6

Ingredients

1 medium onion, chopped

1 tablespoon olive oil

1crushed clove garlic

1/2 teaspoon cumin

1 chopped green capsicum,

1 chopped red capsicum,

2 large chopped carrots,

400g tin chopped tomatoes

2 pints (1.5 litres) of beef stock

½ cup red lentils

1 zucchini, sliced

400g tin drained and rinsed red kidney beans,

1 medium sweet potato, chopped

STEPS;

1. Put the oil, garlic, onion and cumin into a large saucepan.

2. Cook on a medium heat until the onion is softened.

3. Add the carrots, capsicum, tomatoes, lentils, zucchini and stock and bring to the boil.

4. Lower the heat and allow to simmer for about 20 minutes.

5. Add the kidney beans to the saucepan and allow to simmer a further 5 minutes.

6. Let it cool slightly and then pour into a blender and blend.

7. Serve

Hummus

Serves: 6

Ingredients

1 large tin chickpeas, drained and rinsed

1-2 tablespoons tahini paste

2 garlic cloves

Juice of one lemon

STEPS;

1. Blend all the ingredients and if required add more lemon juice

2. Serve as a dip with toasted pita bread or vegetable crudités.

Smoked salmon delights

Serves: 8

Ingredients

20 watercracker biscuits

12 pieces of smoked salmon

120g ricotta cheese

70g cream cheese

1 tspoon capers

1 tspoon lemon juice

lemon zest

1 tspoon spring onions thinly sliced

1 tspoon dill, cut

STEPS;

1 Place the salmon on a platter

2. Put all other ingredients (except biscuits) in a mixing bowl and mix.

3. Place 1 tablespoon of the mixture over on top of each slice of salmon

4. Roll the salmon into a roll

5. Serve with water crackers

Ginger and Carrot salad

Serves: 4

Ingredients

2 tbspoons lightly roasted sesame seeds,

3 carrots thinly sliced

1 cup bean sprouts fresh

Dressing ingredients

½ cup lemon juice fresh

2 dessert spoons sesame oil

3 teaspoons grated ginger- fresh

4 tspoons brown sugar

Black pepper freshly ground

STEPS;

1. Mix all the dressing ingredients together in a bowl and pour over the salad ingredients.

2. Toss well.

Cucumber Salad

Ingredients

Lettuce,

Watercress,

Cucumber,

Tomato,

A small carrot,

Lemon juice,

Fresh mint.

STEPS;

On a base of lettuce and watercress, arrange plenty of thinly sliced cucumber. Decorate with a few wedge of tomato and some grated carrot. Garnish with lemon juice and chopped fresh mint.

Artichoke Salad

Ingredients;

1 large globe artichoke

Crisp lettuce

Bay leaf,

Sprig of thyme

Lemon juice

Olive oil,

Sea Salt

Coriander Seeds

STEPS;

Mix all together in a large bowl

Cabbage, tuna and corn fritters

Ingredients

180g tin tuna in springwater, drained

0.50 cabbage, thinly shredded

tin creamed corn

1 medium onion, finely diced

1/3 cup self raising flour

2 eggs, lightly beaten

0.25 cup reduced fat milk

Olive oil spray

STEPS;

1. Place all ingredients in a bowl, mix well and allow to stand for 15 minutes

2. Blend the mixture in a food processor

3. Heat a frying pan over a low-medium heat and spray with oil

4. Put the mixture in the heated frying pan

5. Fry until golden on both sides

6. Serve with sweet chili sauce

MAIN COURSES

Chilli con carne

Serves: 6

Ingredients

400g lean stewing steak cut into 1 in cubes

1 large onion, sliced

1 carrot sliced

2 crushed garlic clove

1 tin tomatoes chopped

2 tins of kidney beans, well drained

1 packet taco seasoning

Chilli flakes dried

4 tbsps tomato paste

2 beef stock cubes

11/2 tablespoons of olive oil

STEPS;

1. Lightly heat the olive oil and

brown the steak cubes. Set aside

2. Sauté the carrot, onion, garlic and chilli flakes.

3. Place the steak and vegetable mixture in a casserole dish with the taco seasoning, beef stock, chopped tomatoes and tomato paste.

4. Place a lid or cover on the casserole dish and bake in a 180°C oven for approximately 1 ½ hrs.

5. Then mix in the kidney beans and bake for a further 30 minutes.

6. Can be served with brown rice or new potatoes and salad.

Salmon with walnut

Serves: 4-6

Ingredients

2 medium salmon fillets coated with olive oil

1 tablespoon extra olive oil

1/3 cup parsley, cut thinly

1/3 cup dill, cut thinly

2 crushed garlic clove,

1/3 cup roasted dry walnuts crushed

11/2 tablespoons lemon juice

Lemon slices for decoration

STEPS;

Preheat the oven to 180°C

1. Place baking paper in baking dish and place in the oiled salmon and bake for 6 minutes

2. Mix all the crust ingredients together in a bowl.

3. Remove the baking dish from the oven and spread the salmon with ½ of the

crust mixture.

4. Put back into the oven for another 8 to 12 minutes depending on your preference for rare or well cooked.

5. Carefully cut the salmon into 4 to 6 servings and place on a serving plate.

6. Sprinkle with the rest of the crust mixture.

6. Decorate with lemon slices.

Serve with hot new potatoes and a salad

Spinach pie

Serves: 6

Ingredients

1 pkt filo pastry

Olive oil

2 pkts fresh spinach

200g feta cheese, chopped

250g ricotta cheese (low fat)

3 lightly beaten eggs,

2 tblsps fresh dill, cut

3 tblsps fresh mint, cut

8 sliced shallots

1/3 cup of pine-nuts

STEPS;

1. In a bowl, mix the spinach, feta, beaten eggs, ricotta, pine nuts and herbs.

2. Season with salt and freshly ground black pepper.

3. Coat the filo sheets on both sides with olive oil

4. Place half the filo sheets to line a baking dish.

5. Place the spinach, feta, beaten eggs, ricotta, pine nuts and herbs over the pastry and place the remaining filo sheets on top, making sure they are tucked down well around the sides.

6. Bake for 45 minutes in a moderate oven.

7. Stand for 8 minutes before cutting

Serve with a green salad and new potatoes garnished with mint leaves.

Vegetable curry

Serves: 4

Ingredients

4 large potatoes cut into small cubes

2 large sweet potatoes

1 large chopped onion

1cauliflower,

2 carrot, chopped

1 broccoli

4 crushed garlic cloves

3 tsp fresh ginger,

1 1/2 cups vegetable stock

125mls tomato puree

1 cup baby peas frozen

1 tablespoon curry paste

1 cup Greek yoghurt

2 teaspoons cornflour

2 teaspoons chopped mint

Serve with cooked basmati rice

STEPS;

1. In a frying pan heat the oil gently

and add the onions and cook until softened

2. Add the ginger and the garlic and cook, stirring continuously for one minute

3. Add the carrot, cauliflower, potatoes and curry paste.

4. Heat through and stir before adding the tomato puree and vegetable stock

5. Simmer until the vegetables are tender, about 15 mins

6. Stir ½ cup of yoghurt and corn flour into the curry,

7. Add the broccoli and peas.

8. Simmer until all is cooked.

9. Serve with basmati rice and ½ cup of yogurt mixed with mint.

Savoury Rissoles

Ingredients

100g (4oz) cooked butter beans

100g (4oz) milled mixed nuts

50g (2oz) flaked oats

1 egg

1 large onion

2 tomatoes

1 tsp dried sage

½ tsp mixed herbs

Olive oil

Whole-wheat breadcrumbs

Yeast extract

STEPS

Chop the onion and cook in a little oil until soft

Add the mashed beans, nuts, oats, herbs and yeast extract and stir well.

Add the beaten egg and the tomatoes chopped.

Adjust seasoning to taste.

Shape into four equal sized rissoles, place on baking sheet,

Brush with oil and sprinkle with breadcrumbs.

Cook in moderate oven 177C/350F (Gas Mark 4) for approx 30 minutes, until nicely browned and crisp on top.

Chicken risotto

Serves: 4-6

Ingredients

1 onion, chopped

1/2 tablespoon olive oil

1 teaspoon minced garlic

400g chicken breast cubed

2 cups rice

5 cups salt-reduced chicken stock

2½ cups button mushrooms, sliced

1 small floret broccoli

1/4 cup white wine

Pepper to season

2 cups baby spinach leaves

STEPS;

1. In a frying pan cook the onion and garlic in the oil over low-medium heat until softened

2. Add the chicken and stir until browned.

3. Add the rice and stir for 5 minutes, until the rice has changed colour slightly

4. Add the wine and stir until absorbed

5. Add 1 cup of stock and stir until absorbed

6. Add the broccoli, spinach and another cup of stock, stir until absorbed

7. Add the mushrooms and the remaining 2 cups of stock, one at a time – making sure the liquid has been absorbed before adding more

8. Cook until rice is ready

9. Remove from the heat, season with pepper and serve.

Easy Tarragon Chicken

Ingredients;

1 Chicken

2 tbsps unsalted butter

1 tbsp chopped fresh tarragon

1 clove garlic, chopped

Sea salt and black pepper

Olive oil

Steps;

Preheat oven to 200°C

Clean and trim chicken

Mix together the butter, tarragon, garlic and seasoning

Place the mixture into the cavity of the chicken secure with a cocktail stick

Rub the skin of the chicken with olive oil.

Place the chicken upside down in a roasting tin and toast for 1 ¼-1 ½ hours basting at intervals.

Serve with a mixed green salad and a

vegetable of your choice lightly steamed.

DESSERTS

Custard with Baked apples

Serves: 4

Ingredients

4 apples

1/2 cup chopped walnuts,

4 tblesps syrup

1 tblesps water

1 dessert spoon margerine

1 tspoon cinnamon

Custard ingredients

600 mls low-fat milk

2 tblsps cornflour

1 tblsps sugar

2 slightly beaten egg yolks,

1/3 tspoon extract of vanilla

STEPS;

---

1. Clean apples and remove cores

2. Insert small cuts in the apples at the bottom and top.

3. In a small bowl mix together the cinnamon sultanas and walnuts,

4. In the space where the cores were fill with the nut and fruit mix.

5. Inside each apple pour 1 tablespoon of syrup.

6. Put the apples in a baking dish with the water and margarine.

7. Bake covered until the apples are softened (approximately30 minutes.)

8. While the apples are cooking prepare the custard by heating nearly all the milk in a pan.

9. Blend the remaining milk with the sugar and corn-flour until smooth.

10. Add in the beaten egg yolks

11. Shortly before the milk boils, remove from the heat and add in the corn flour mixture. Stir.

12. Keep stirring back on the heat until the mixture thickens and boils.

13. Simmer stirring continuously until the custard is thoroughly cooked.

14. Remove from the heat and mix in the vanilla extract

15. Pour into a dish and keep covered until ready to serve.

Apple crumble

Serves: 6

Ingredients

8 medium apples, cored, peeled, and chopped

11/4 tblesp sugar

2 tablsps water

2 tsps margarine

2 tablsps honey

1 cup oats

1 tsp cinnamon

1/3 cup sultanas

1/2 cup plain flour

STEPS

1. Warm oven to 170°C

2. Place water, sugar and apples in a covered saucepan, and cook until softened.

3. Put the apple mixture into an ovenproof baking dish

4. Mix the margarine and honey in a saucepan and heat gently until melted.

5. Then pour onto the flour, oats, and cinnamon and stir until well mixed.

6. Put the crumble mixture on top of the apples and bake for approximately 25 minutes until it becomes golden.

7. Serve hot with cream or custard.

RECAP;

To lessen the liver's workload, it is advisable to follow a diet that is low in fats, alcohol and sugars, and to cut down on tea and coffee. Remember the liver is your friend. Take care of it.

If you enjoyed this book, please leave a review.

LOVE YOUR LIVER:How to keep your liver healthy (HEALTHY LIVING)

OTHER BOOKS BY THIS AUTHOR

FISH AND SEAFOOD FOR LOVE (NATURE'S NATURAL APRODISIACS)

The ancient world believed seafood had aphrodisiac characteristics because, the Greek goddess of love, Aphrodite, sprang from the foam of the sea on an oyster shell (hence Botticelli's much reproduced painting of the goddess floating on a seashell). The Romans named her Venus.

The sea is one of the major sources of life and Seafood has been seen as the food of love for many centuries. A claim that is not surprising considering it is brimming with minerals such as calcium, zinc, iodine and iron.

In this delightful book of aphrodisiac foods, the author looks at the most popular fishy aphrodisiacs as well as providing some excellent recipes to enjoy them.

HERBS AND SPICES FOR LOVE: ENHANCE YOUR SEX LIFE (Nature's Natural Aphrodisiacs Book 1)

Enhance your diet with the use of natural herbs and spices and improve your love life.

According to Greek mythology, Aphrodite - the goddess of love, beauty, fertility and desire had emerged from the waters carrying some herbs with her. The plants she brought had powers to excite sexual desire, and came to be known as aphrodisiacs.

The heady aromas and flavors of expensive, exotic spices have been known since ancient times to create a "stimulating" environment. Every ancient culture testifies to the sexually stimulating properties of certain foods. Herbs included;